Quick123

• GUIDES TO EVERYTHING •

Food for THOUGHT

Good NUTRITION for HEALTHY Kids

By Cora Lydon

ISBN 978-1-84678-005-9

Quick123 Limited, PO Box 45092, London N4 2ZJ.

Website: www.quick123.co.uk

Customer service or additional copies can be sought at service@quick123.co.uk.

Letter to the Reader

Children are notoriously fussy eaters. There's many a child who has survived on a diet of fish fingers and jam sandwiches, despite the best efforts of its parents to provide a healthy and nutritious diet.

This shows that a bad diet is rarely fatal in itself. I myself was an incredibly fussy child who refused just about all the major food groups and lived on a diet of chicken and potatoes. And, yes, I made it to adulthood with no apparent scars.

Even so, it is in these early years that the habits of a lifetime are set. Those habits will have a big impact on health, fitness and well-being in the years to come.

At least 8.5 per cent of six year olds and 15 per cent of 15 year olds in the United Kingdom are thought to be obese. That doesn't even include the number of children who are overweight.

With this obesity epidemic sweeping the country, it is more important than ever to get children into good eating habits as early as possible.

Of course, it's all very well knowing that children should be eating a healthy, balanced diet, but what does it really involve and how on earth are you going to convince them? I hope you will discover from this guide that it needn't be the battleground that you might imagine.

Yes, at times it will be difficult and yes, you can expect tears and tantrums – but follow the suggestions in these pages and I'm convinced that you'll be well on the road to success.

Cora Lydon

Contents

Quick123 GUIDES TO EVERYTHING

Quick123 Limited
PO Box 45092
London N4 2ZJ

Email: peterpurton@quick123.co.uk

Dear Quick123 reader

Thank you for buying this guide. We hope you enjoy reading it.

Our aim is to help you achieve the goals you set yourself, whether it's getting a better job, improving relationships or creating a better you. And to help you achieve that without costing you too much time, effort or money.

Because you, the reader, are at the centre of everything we do, we'd like to hear from you. Whether you have comments about this book, ideas for a new topic or issues in your life you feel we might be able to help with, send us an email or a letter.

If we take up any of your ideas to create a new title we'll make sure you get your own special copy.

We want to provide you with the kinds of guides you want to read. With your help, I'm sure we can.

Happy reading,

Peter Purton

Peter Purton
Quick123 Limited

The importance of healthy eating

We all know that healthy eating is important in helping to stave off illness and keeping our bodies in optimum working condition. This becomes all the more obvious when it comes to feeding your offspring.

The scale of growth and development in the first few years of life is incredible. By the age of two, you can expect the weight of your once-tiny bundle of joy to have tripled or in some cases even quadrupled.

It doesn't stop there: most teenagers show a growth spurt during puberty. The main ingredient needed to support these changes is of course food – and, more to the point, a healthy, balanced diet.

The Royal College of Psychiatrists believes that a third of under-fives are suffering from some form of mild to moderate eating problem. This may lead them to refuse some or all of those foods that are known for their ability to help with proper growth and development.

Short-term fussiness about food is to be expected in most children. However, if this behaviour develops into a long-term problem, it could be responsible for stunting their development.

Over the past decade, children's poor eating habits have become one of the most discussed topics in the UK, yet the problem still persists. It is important to encourage your child in a healthy eating regime but without restricting their food intake.

If your child is overweight, it is essential not to put them on a specific weight-reduction programme that may do more harm than good. Aside from making your child feel self-conscious about their weight (which they may not have seen as an issue previously) it can also lead to deficiencies in vital nutrients.

Seek advice

Seek advice from your GP to help you devise a balanced eating plan. Remember, it is important to keep your child at a healthy weight.

A recent Commons select committee report found that obesity levels in children had more than tripled between 1994 and 2002. If this trend continues, today's children will be the first for more than a century whose life expectancy is lower than that of their parents.

Many children are left to their own devices and wield too much control over their parents and dinner menus. It's rare to see a child opt for a piece of fruit rather than a bag of crisps, for example.

Sometimes striking the right balance can be tricky. You want to train their taste buds – while allowing them some degree of freedom – and get them to eat enough nutritious foods to keep them healthy.

It can be done, with some gentle persuasion, a bit of effort on your part and an understanding of what children really need.

TOP TIPS

10 tips for a healthy diet

1. A varied diet will give your child the best chance of obtaining all of the nutrients they need to be healthy. Make time to experiment with new ingredients. If they don't like jacket potato, try them with potato wedges or mashed potato. Children are often quite conscious of different textures, so persevere.

2. Beware of their liquid consumption. Many of the drinks we offer our children are calorie-dense but nutrient-poor. Good choices include water, milk, smoothies and fruit juices diluted with water. Fizzy drinks, even low cal varieties, should be avoided: most contain e-numbers and far too much sugar.

3. Never use food as a reward for good behaviour, or withhold it for bad behaviour. Instead, try a trip to the park, a small gift from the toyshop or books and CDs for older kids as incentives.

4. Try to make sure that they are eating at least five portions of fruit and vegetables daily. Always offer them fruit as a snack and keep your fruit bowl piled high to tempt them.

5. Make sure they always start the day with a nourishing and healthy breakfast to keep them fuelled till lunch. Try porridge with berries in winter and fresh fruit and muesli in summer.

6. If you can afford to go for organic then do so. These foods are unlikely to contain any pesticide residue and the organic regulations prohibit the use of any synthetic colourings and flavourings.

7. Avoid buying foods that have been produced with children in mind. There is absolutely no harm in your child eating the same food as the rest of your family, and at least you can be sure that it is wholesome.

8. Keep an eye on their portion sizes. Most children do not have the same appetite as adults so don't pile their plates too high. If they are still hungry, offer extra vegetables or salad to bulk a meal out.

9. Stay calm when faced with a child steadfastly refusing to eat. Don't offer to make another dish; suggest they leave the table and return when they are ready to eat. Children are unlikely to starve themselves: they will eat something if they are hungry.

10. Don't add salt to children's food or keep a salt cellar on the table. Allow children's taste buds to develop without overloading on salt. You can liven up dishes through using herbs, oils or spices.

Did You Know... ?

- Lack of calcium (found in dairy products and leafy green vegetables) can hamper the formation of healthy bones

- A deficiency of vitamin A (sourced from carrots and other highly coloured fruit and vegetables) can harm their eyesight

What every child needs

The National Diet and Nutrition Survey in 2000 contained some revealing statistics about children's eating habits. One in ten four to six year olds ate no green leafy vegetables whatsoever; fewer than one in 25 reached the recommended five portions of fruit and vegetables.

Over a seven-day period, 80 per cent of young people consumed white bread, savoury snacks, pickles, savoury sauces, gravies, condiments, crisps, biscuits and chocolates. Offering them healthy choices and not banning foods may be the key to improving their diet.

Remember, it is important to place everything in context. When we talk about a balanced diet, we should be considering diet over a few days or a week.

If you discover that their lunch money has been spent on a bag of chips and a can of pop, don't panic – it can be balanced with a home-cooked meal loaded with vegetables.

As a general rule, a balanced diet for children would include food from each of the following food groups:

- Fruit and vegetables
  (aim for at least five portions a day)
- Bread, other cereals or potatoes (with every meal)
- Milk and dairy foods
  (two to three servings a day)
- Meat, fish and alternatives
  (one to two lean servings a day)
- Foods containing fat and sugar
  (in limited amounts)

A balanced menu for children over five should contain the right balance of nutrients – 45 per cent carbs (carbohydrates), 20 per cent protein and no more than 35 per cent fat.

Carbs: this covers bread, rice, pasta and other cereals. Carbs are the body's main source of energy and also have a good supply of iron – which is vital for energy, intellectual performance and good health.

"A balanced menu for children over five should contain the right balance of nutrients – 45 per cent carbs (carbohydrates), 20 per cent protein and no more than 35 per cent fat"

Try to opt for wholegrain options rather than white varieties. Wholegrain versions release sugar more slowly into the bloodstream. This provides longer lasting energy. Refined carbs, such as white bread, pasta and rice, have also lost many of their nutrients in their processing.

Fruit and vegetables: Fruit and vegetables are vital for good health: they provide phytochemicals, which can protect against cancer. They are also a good source of fibre, while root vegetables are excellent starchy carbs.

To tempt kids, you may need to do more than just serve up some boiled carrots. Try giving them corn on the cob, which most kids love to nibble on, or adding it to sauces and pasta or rice dishes. Vegetables that are steamed retain more of their nutrients than those that are boiled to death!

Dairy: As well as being one of the best sources of calcium, dairy products provide protein, vitamins and minerals. They are also important for healthy bones and teeth. Young children should not be given low fat food, as they need the full fat varieties for energy and growth. Give them milk to drink, a yoghurt to snack on or cheese with lunch.

Protein: This is essential for the growth, maintenance and repair of body tissue. Not getting enough can reduce children's resistance to infection. Meat, poultry, fish, pulses, eggs and nuts are all good sources. Oily fish is an excellent choice as it contains essential fatty acids which are used by the body for the formation of bones and ligaments and are important for brain growth.

A healthy diet should also be one that minimises 'negative' nutrients – those that, in unhealthy proportions, only serve to promote ill-health. The three main nutrients that this can be applied to are:

Saturated fat: This is found in butter, margarine, fatty meat, processed foods and cheese. Always use meat products that have a high meat content (80 per cent or more), or switch to lean meat. Use spreads and oils sparingly.

Salts: Foods high in salt include savoury snacks like crisps, convenience foods and packet foods. Always read the labels of foods so you know exactly how much salt a product contains. Cut back on processed and convenience foods and never add salt to meals or have it at the table.

Processed sugars: Some sugars that occur naturally, such as those found in fruit, are better for your child than processed sugars, which are found in soft drinks, puddings, biscuits, sweets and chocolates. Instead of offering puddings, tempt them with fruit, and always give them water and milk to drink in place of fizzy drinks and squashes.

Did You Know...
A study undertaken by Cancer Research UK showed children and their parents tend to eat similar quantities of fresh fruit and vegetables

With obesity sweeping the country, there's never been a better time to focus on your child's diet. Being obese or even mildly overweight can have a profound effect on your child's life. The emotional issues include bullying and lack of self-confidence.

Being classed as obese may shave as many as nine years off your child's life. Conditions such as heart disease, type 2 diabetes, high blood pressure and osteoarthritis are all common chronic ailments linked to carrying extra pounds.

How diet affects children

Consumption of too much junk food can have dire consequences for your children's behaviour. It has always been suspected that artificial food colourings can affect children's mood and behaviour. Scientific studies are now beginning to back the idea.

A government-funded study conducted by the Asthma & Allergy Research Centre in 2002 concluded that all children could benefit from the removal of artificial food colourings from their diet. The study was conducted on 227 three year olds.

It tested the effects of a drink that contained food colourings at a level below the current permitted level, and a preservative at the permitted level. The parents involved reported significant changes in their children's behaviour, such as temper tantrums and fidgeting.

Many additives have already been banned in other countries, for example, the US, Sweden and Denmark, while still being classed as safe in the UK. There is plenty of anecdotal advice that suggests we are getting it wrong in the UK.

Some experts believe that the impact on behaviour is due to the fact that additives prevent

"It is recognised that a lack of zinc is a factor in hyperactivity"

the body from absorbing as much zinc as it should from foods. It is recognised that a lack of zinc is a factor in hyperactivity.

In comparison, a diet that is balanced, nutritious and rich in fruit and vegetables helps promote good health in your children. It will help with their growth and development in their formative years. It should also lay down good health habits for the future and help protect them from a wide range of ailments and diseases.

"Consumption of too much junk food can have dire consequences for your children's behaviour"

Wise Words

It stands to reason that any food that hasn't been processed or 'fiddled about with' in some way has to be better for your child than what has emerged from a production line. Think natural, and you should be on the right lines!

Six main food fads

According to Dr David Lewis, a psychologist who has studied children and food, there are six main food fads that children go through:

ANGER FADS

This is particularly common in children who have yet to master an understanding of language. Food may be refused to express their anger.

Get it right: Identify and remove the cause of their anger. Encourage them to communicate through other means (such as baby signing).

INDEPENDENCE FADS

As children start to get older, they like to assert their independence and one easy way is to reject food that mum and dad want them to eat.

Get it right: Let them be independent in other areas, such as choosing what they wear or what they will play with.

COPYCAT FADS

The bigger your brood, the more likely you are to have to deal with this one. Children revel in copying each other's (often poor) eating habits.

Get it right: Children want you to react, so ignore their behaviour and it should settle down. Make sure that they always have the opportunity to watch mum and dad eat and make sure your diet is healthy.

ANXIETY FADS

As children grow up, they also begin to understand more about the world around them. Some may start to associate chicken with the film *Chicken Run* and bacon with *Babe*.

Get it right: Never force them to eat a particular food, which can make the situation worse. Look for alternatives you can offer them which still give them plenty of nutrients. With time the anxiety should fade.

STRANGE FOOD FADS

Most children are pre-programmed to be wary of strange foods, so they may not try them without a fight.

Get it right: Keep offering the dish to them every few weeks, and let them see how much you enjoy it. If they're still not keen you can always try preparing the dish in another way.

ALLERGY FADS

Rather impressively, some children know instinctively that a certain food will make them physically ill and so will avoid it.

Get it right: Never force food onto children if they have a strong objection to it. Look for alternatives.

Get them to love the foods they hate!

Sometimes it's necessary to resort to stealth tactics to sneak some goodness into their diet:

- When making sauces for pasta or cooking minced meat, add finely chopped vegetables and they'll never even know they're there!

- Think about the presentation – something that looks tasty will more often than not entice them to try at least one mouthful.

- Get them involved with food preparation and cooking. It's always much more interesting to eat something that you've cooked yourself.

- Use spices, herbs, a drizzle of oil or lemon juice to add some flavour to the meal.

- A fruit smoothie is always appreciated by youngsters and contains a healthy dose of goodness! However, because juiced fruit loses its fibre content you should also ensure they are eating some fresh fruit too.

- Sit down as a family so that your child gets used to seeing other people enjoying food.

- Mash root vegetables (swede, sweet potato, carrots etc) together to create a tasty, nutrient-rich mash.

- Try a change of scenery! When the weather's right you might be able to encourage them to eat some fruit and vegetables if they can eat their meal in the Wendy house, for example!

- Don't expect little kids to eat adult-sized portions, but serve up smaller family meals. Your child may refuse to eat if they feel daunted by the sheer volume of food that has been served up to them.

- If they don't like jacket potatoes, try giving them mash, wedges or roast potatoes. More often than not, all it takes is a change in texture.

- Peer pressure can work wonders, so let them invite a friend round for tea who you know likes eating healthily. Just watch as they copy their friend's behaviour.

Food labelling

Nowadays, you need to have a degree in food nutrition to decipher what the labels on your food packaging actually mean. Manufacturers are keen to highlight 'added vitamins' while burying the high salt, fat and calorie contents of their foods.

To make sure that you are feeding your children good, healthy, nutritious foods, you need to become a bit of a food detective. You'll need to read between the lines.

While you may think that food labels can actually make your job as chief nutritionist easier, the opposite can be true. More and more manufacturers are jumping on the healthy-eating bandwagon and plastering packets of crisps, chocolates and pizza with outlandish health claims in a bid to lure you in.

Just because that pizza is spread with 'lycopene-rich tomato sauce' and topped with 'cancer-fighting vegetables' doesn't automatically make it a healthy choice. Your food choices should be focussed on the overall healthiness of the product. That means checking out the salt, fat and calorie content.

It's not illegal for companies to make spurious claims on their packaging. If you're a busy mum with a screaming toddler hanging off your arm, the chances are you don't have the time to investigate the claims further.

When it comes to baby food there *are* certain rules and regulations that manufacturers have to comply with, such as keeping within the maximum permitted levels of sucrose, salt and pesticides. Once your child reaches the age of one, however, these guidelines no longer apply.

These strict guidelines are used to protect babies' health. Their immature livers and kidneys are just not able to cope with the demands of processing some substances.

Just because your child has reached the age of one does not mean that they are now automatically able to process high levels of salt and additives, however. It's important to keep a watchful eye on their diet.

"By law, all food packaging must show ingredients, genetically-modified ingredients, nutritional information and any artificial sweeteners the foodstuffs contain"

By law, all foods must show certain information on their labelling. Packaging should show ingredients, genetically-modified ingredients, nutritional information and any artificial sweeteners the foodstuffs contain.

Look at the ingredients

Just how do you go about interpreting this information? The first thing to do is to take a look at the ingredients list. The ingredients making up your food will be written in descending order of weight.

You may not even recognise some of the names. Many manufacturers are guilty of using alternative names for certain items.

Despite the unfamiliar names, it is surprising how many mums and dads would feel safer letting their children consume glucose, fructose, maltose, dextrose, fruit syrup or molasses than ordinary sugar. In fact they are all the same thing.

In order to get an idea of the total sugar content you need to look on the nutritional panel and read 'carbohydrates – of which sugar...'.

Basic guidelines

The government has published some basic guidelines that can be used to judge how healthy your shopping is. Copy or cut out the panel opposite and take it to the supermarket with you:

A lot	Nutrient	A little
10g	Sugars	2g
20g	Fat	3g
5g	Saturated fat	1g
3g	Fibre	0.5g
0.5g	Sodium	0.1g

Salt

Our tastes as adults are directly influenced by our childhood diets, so making sure that your children stick to a healthy level of salt is a great idea. As a nation we are eating far too much of it.

"Children are not born with an innate liking for salt - the preference is developed throughout their early years"

Salt does have a vital role to play in our diets; even so, too much can lead to high blood pressure and hypertension. Children are not born with an innate liking for salt – the preference is developed throughout their early years.

In the UK it is estimated that a whopping 75 per cent of salt consumed comes from processed foods, takeaways, sweets, snacks and meals bought and consumed outside the home. When it comes to your own children, you should avoid adding any salt to their cooking or at the table, and try to reduce the amount of processed food they eat. But beware, salt can be found in the unlikeliest of places, such as bread and cheese.

To work out the salt content of a product that doesn't list it clearly, just multiply the listed sodium content by 2.5 to get a rough estimate.

The government's Scientific Advisory Committee on Nutrition has issued the following targets for children's salt intake:

Age	Salt target (g/day)
0-6 months	Less than 1g
7-12 months	1g
1-3 years	2g
4-6 years	3g
7-10 years	5g
11-14 years	6g

GM ingredients

Many people are suspicious of genetically modified ingredients. The fact is that, as yet, we do not know the risks that may be involved with eating them on a regular basis.

As they are a relatively new concept, it is likely to be a while before people become aware of any possible side effects they may have. They may not even have any.

"Labelling does not need to point out the milk and animal products that have been derived from animals fed with genetically modified feed"

At present, in Europe, packaging must display the fact that a food is genetically modified. Even so, there are some loopholes.

Food that unintentionally contains less than one per cent of genetically modified material does not need to be labelled. The same goes for food that is produced from genetically modified plants but does not contain genetically modified material.

Labelling does not need to point out the products that have been derived from animals fed with genetically modified feed. So, although you may think you are avoiding GM foods, food can be produced with the help of genetic engineering – and the packaging need not say so.

Additives and E numbers

You should also look out for artificial colourings, additives and preservatives on packaging. Most of the regulatory data that has been collected on additives and their safety has been compiled from studies conducted on adults. Yet children's immune and excretory systems do not work at the same capacity as adults'.

When it comes to E-numbers, many of the most common offenders are likely to be found in the very food loved by children. Manufacturers have also found ways of getting round the fact that their product contains additives.

For instance, most parents can pick up an item and look out for ingredients such as E211 and E124. How many would be able to spot sodium benzoate or ponceau 4R as additives, though? As manufacturers have picked up on parents getting wise to E-number labelling, the labels have started to change.

"There is nothing to stop manufacturers using flavour enhancers in products eaten by young children"

Some flavour enhancers, such as monosodium glutamate, are banned from foods aimed at children under three. Despite this, there is nothing to stop manufacturers using them in products that may not be aimed at young children, but are most certainly eaten by them.

If in doubt, always avoid food that is highly coloured. Try to familiarise yourself with some of the most common food additives and flavourings used.

The following table is by no means exhaustive but will provide a starting point for detecting artificial ingredients in your children's food.

E number	Name	Use	Possible harmful side effects
E951	Aspartame	Sweetener	Carcinogenic, hyperactivity
E210	Benzoic acid	Preservative	Asthma, rhinitis, urticaria
E621	Monosodium glutamate	Flavour enhancer	Headaches, nausea, asthma
E308	Phosphoric acid	Food additive	Excessive consumption can lead to loss of bone calcium
E102	Tartrazine	Colouring	Hyperactivity, asthma, rhinitis, urticaria
E290	Carbon dioxide	Fizz and preservative	Long term use reduces fertility

Food labelling is strictly governed by law. That doesn't stop many manufacturers making their products sound a whole lot better than they really are.

It all comes down to knowing what certain terms and words mean. For example:

- A food can only claim to be reduced calorie if it is much lower in calories than the usual version. This does not necessarily mean that it is a low calorie choice

- 'Low fat', 'low sodium', 'reduced salt' and 'high fibre' arc all general enough claims. They may sound good but mean little. There are no legal definitions for quantities (except for butter, margarine and other spreadable fats)

- The words 'lite' or 'light' also have no legal definition. They don't mean that your choice of food is going to be any healthier

- When it comes to fat, claims recommendations have been put forward by the Food Standards Agency. 'Low fat' should only be used in foods that contain less then three grams of fat per 100g, while 'fat free' should be used only when a food contains less than 0.15g per 100g

- Don't be fooled by the words 'natural', 'made from natural' or 'pure'; all it means is that the manufacturer started with a natural source. The product itself can still be processed

- Don't automatically assume that organic means a food is healthy. It does limit the number of pesticides used but it may still be just as unhealthy as a regular version of the same product

"When it comes to deciphering the labelling of products, the best rule of thumb is to read the ingredients list and nutrition panel and ignore the claims made on the front"

When it comes to deciphering the labelling of products, the best rule of thumb is to read the ingredients list and nutrition panel and ignore the claims made on the front.

Look out for a long list of ingredients with names that are hard to pronounce (they are most likely to be artificial ingredients). Instead, go for products that sound all together more tempting and wholesome.

Real appeal

When it comes to buying food for your children, be aware of some of the methods that manufacturers use to sell you that food. For example, have you ever noticed how:

Many desserts are now topped with sweets? This is a common ploy to draw kids in. Sweets have little, if any, nutritional value and only add more e-numbers.

Celebrities or cartoon characters are used to endorse products? Those savvy manufacturers know what kids want. If it's got their hero plastered over it, you can bet they'll want it.

How products vie with each other to be different? Take bread, for example. No longer do you just have the choice of white or wholemeal, now you can have white bread with the added goodness of wholemeal and even crustless slices!

Coronation Street is sandwiched between endless adverts for kids' food? The whole aim of any advert is to increase a product's pulling power.

Nowhere is it more apparent than with products aimed at kids.

At first glance the product seems more than acceptable? This is one of the hardest traps for parents to avoid. Manufacturers know it is parents who make the decisions and so do their best to make it appeal to the buyer by using claims of healthy nutrition.

Wise Words

The more you read the information given to you on packaging, the more you will start to wise up to what's actually in there and to read between the lines. Remember that it's in the manufacturers' interest to sell you their product!

Get into good eating habits

It's all very well expecting your children to eat a healthy, balanced diet. If you yourself don't act as a good role model, where can you expect them to pick up their good eating habits from?

Children love to copy what they see: young girls will care for dolls the way they see mum looking after a younger sibling; young boys will imitate scenes from their favourite hero cartoons. It is your responsibility to make sure that you set a good example.

We like to think we are giving them the very best start to a healthy life. Even those parents who regularly consume plenty of fruit and vegetables at the dinner table can still get it wrong.

Habits that are developed in childhood more often than not continue into adulthood. Then it's easy to see how a life of unhealthy eating habits lies ahead.

Some of the key traps that adults fall into are easy to put right. You just need to be able to identify them first.

Not eating breakfast

Although the message is starting to filter through, there are still many parents who believe they are far too busy to eat the most important meal of the day.

Why is it so important? If a child eats its final meal of the day at about 5pm (as many children do) and then has nothing to eat until the next day, it is quite possible for them to go for up to 18 hours without breaking that fast.

This lack of food does nothing to help their concentration or behaviour, so it's important to get into good breakfasting habits as early as possible. Each morning, offer your children some muesli or porridge or scrambled eggs on toast.

Avoid sugar-coated cereals which will cause an energy burst that will tail off within an hour or two and leave them lacklustre. If you need to, set the alarm a few minutes early to make sure you have time to sit and eat breakfast with them.

"it's important to get into good breakfasting habits as early as possible"

You can even do all the preparation before you go to bed the night before.

Bribery

What parent hasn't resorted to underhand methods of enticing their child to behave, eat their greens or go to school? In the long term these methods will only backfire.

If you limit unhealthy choices but then offer items such as ice cream or sweets as a reward, this bribery will only leave your children confused. Instead, make sure that no food is banned, but always explain to them the nutrient and health values of the food you *do* offer. Your children will then begin to make healthy choices for themselves. Banning food is only more likely to make them want it. As they grow up, they may indulge in this food just because they can – and you won't be there to supervise.

If you are looking for a way to reward them, avoid food bribes altogether. Instead, offer a visit to the swimming pool or a new toy.

Pre-conception and pregnancy diet

Although your diet during this time may not have a direct impact on your child's future diet, it can have a direct effect on their health.

The chances of having healthy offspring are much better when both you and your partner are in the prime of health. It may take a few months prior to conception to achieve this.

Experts believe that poor nutrition before and during a pregnancy can lead to a child not achieving its full potential. It's certainly worth considering that, if you are short of essential nutrients during your early pregnancy, the baby may not have all that it needs to develop well.

Breastfeeding

What if we were to tell you that there *is* a way to get your kids to like vegetables? Great, we hear you yell – but it may be you've already missed the boat with your kids.

"If you eat a wide variety of foods while feeding your infant then you can hope that your child will be more open to eating a wide range of foods as they grow up"

It's not just a myth that the flavour of breast milk depends on what you eat. This may be the key to getting them to eat those greens.

This theory is supported by the fact that babies of different cultures have different tastes. A baby from a traditional Indian family will happily embrace the spicy flavours of a curry if it was introduced to them in their breast milk.

If you eat a wide variety of foods while feeding your infant then you can hope that your child will be more open to eating a wide range of foods as they grow up.

Dieting

Research from the human nutrition department of Glasgow Royal Hospital for Sick Children has uncovered the worrying fact that children as young as three may be driven towards a life of obesity and eating disorders by their diet-obsessed parents.

The nutritionists involved in the research found that the children of parents who were dieting or over-anxious about food had an increased risk of developing weight problems themselves. Eating disorder specialist, Dr Steve Bratman, believes that a growing number of children are eating such an extremely limited amount of key nutrients that they may be damaging their health.

It's essential that young children are not subjected to the same eating regime as a dieting parent. Children under the age of five need more fat than older children.

Adults need 35 per cent fat, children aged one to three need approximately 42 per cent, kids aged four to five need 40 per cent, while babies need 50 per cent.

Vegetarianism

There is nothing wrong with bringing up your children as vegetarians as long as you ensure that they are getting adequate nutrients to thrive.

One key nutrient that is obtained from red meat is iron. Vegetarians can obtain this from leafy green veg, egg yolks and dried fruits – but not many kids are willing to eat them.

Iron deficiency has dire consequences for long-term health, including anaemia and a lowered IQ. It is thought to affect one in four infants at some point.

Even not getting quite enough iron can hamper your child's progress. It can lead to a decreased appetite, lethargy, developmental delays and behavioural problems.

Most parents are not aware that one of the main causes of iron deficiency in very small children is the introduction of cow's milk as the primary drink in the first year of life. For this reason, mothers should opt for breastfeeding or use an iron-fortified formula.

"Not getting quite enough iron can hamper your child's progress"

Family meals

The death of the family meal has also had dramatic consequences on children's behaviour towards food. Eating together as a family has been shown to instil in children a greater awareness about food and it encourages them to make healthy choices.

Although time may not always allow it, try to eat together as a family at least every other day, even just for dinner. The whole experience of eating together means kids are getting a healthy, home-cooked dinner as well as subconsciously picking up on other people's eating habits.

"Eating together as a family encourages children to make healthy choices"

Interestingly, one study found that having even one parent present during a child's evening meal meant that they were more likely to eat breakfast the next day.

Wise Words

If you are obsessed with dieting, the likelihood is that you will pass the obsession on to your children. Always remember that you are likely to be the best role model they have. If they see you agitating over food issues, the area is likely to get out of proportion in their lives too.

Eating should be a pleasurable pastime, not a war zone for any reason

Ideas for lunchboxes

School dinners have taken a bit of a bashing of late. Sending your children off to school with a packed lunch may be the sensible option. It gives you direct control over what they eat and you can rest assured that they are getting something healthy *and* something they like.

Variety really is the spice of life. By offering them different options you can inspire them to try something new.

A survey of over 550 children's lunchboxes by the Food Standards Agency revealed that nine out of ten contained foods that were too high in saturated fat, salt and sugar. Read on for some top tips.

The ideal lunchbox should be made up of:

Bread/cereals

Don't just give them two slices of white bread. If it's sandwiches they want, then try them with multigrain or wholemeal bread. It needn't stop there! Pitta breads, bagels, Scotch pancakes, fruit scones, rice salads and pasta are all good lunch-time fillers.

Fruit and vegetables

Add salad to sandwiches and rolls; cut up bite sized pieces of fruit; make vegetable *crudités* with a yoghurt dip; add chopped vegetables to pasta; give them dried fruit – it all helps.

Meat, fish and alternatives

Try to offer them something different each day (either as a filling in a roll or sandwich or in a pasta or rice dish). Some good ideas include chicken, turkey, boiled eggs, tuna and quorn slices.

Dairy foods

Children need a good supply of calcium for adequate growth. Offer them a carton of milk, a cheese triangle, a yoghurt or cottage cheese.

If they can't tolerate dairy products, look for other calcium-rich options such as salmon or green leafy vegetables. You can also replace dairy products with soya products.

"When it comes to getting children to eat healthy food, presentation is key"

Liquids

Beware of the empty calories that many drinks aimed at children may contain. High-cal, low-nutrient fizzy drinks should be out. Replace them with milk, fruit smoothies, fruit juice diluted with water or just with plain water itself.

When it comes to getting children to eat healthy food, presentation is key. Get them involved in choosing what they would like to eat (within reason) and encourage them to help you make it. Remember other factors. Most children want to eat their lunch as quickly as possible so they can get out in the playground.

Peel and segment fruit beforehand and offer easy-eating vegetable sticks. If it's going to take them a while to prepare it at school before they can eat it, most kids won't make the effort.

Of course it is all too easy for children not to eat their lunch and for you to be none the wiser. Keep in contact with the school as much as possible to determine that your children are getting enough food each day.

Did You Know... ?

- **Every year more than 5.5 million lunchboxes are packed for children in the UK**
- **The 2004 Lunchbox Survey revealed that ham was the most popular sandwich filler (27 per cent) while white bread was favoured over wholegrain options (69 per cent)**

Could the right food make your kid brainier?

In a word yes – and not only brainier but also better behaved, stronger and with better eyesight! "The key thing about children is that they are not mini-adults," says Lizzie Vann, creator of Organix organic baby foods and the Goodies range of additive-, preservative- and GM-free snacks.

"Their bodies are developing, and all the important systems that have to last life-long are being created – cardiovascular, immune, reproductive, nervous systems, etc. So getting the nutrition wrong during the first ten years of life will cause problems."

Top foods for healthy children

Nuts and seeds: Nuts and seeds are a great snack to give to children as they are extremely nutritious and rich in zinc. Zinc is an essential nutrient. Without it, children can lose their sense of taste and smell and demand ever stronger tastes, which are often created artificially.

> **"Nuts and seeds are a great snack to give to children as they are extremely nutritious and rich in zinc"**

Sprinkle pumpkin seeds or sunflower seeds into porridge or muesli or give them a handful of nuts between meals. Nuts should not be given to children under five or a child who has a nut allergy.

Oily fish: Opt for a good quality oily fish. Research shows that, the more good quality foods you introduce to your child at a young age, the lower the likelihood of their being fussy eaters as they grow up.

Oil-rich fish is essential for the development of the brain and nervous system. Numerous studies have highlighted the many health benefits it offers. Try fish pie, fish kebabs or fishcakes to tempt a fussy eater.

Research has also suggested that a diet that is rich in fatty acids, such as those from oily fish, could improve the performance of children who have dyslexia, dyspraxia and attention deficit disorder.

Red meat: Red meat is one of the best sources of iron, but always try to opt for lean cuts of meat. Also try peas, beans, dried fruits and seeds.

Lack of iron means children lose motivation and interest in what is going on around them, struggle to concentrate and lose the ability to get up and be active. Beef chilli, shepherd's pie and lentil soup are all good iron-rich choices.

Porridge: Researchers have found that children who eat a breakfast with a low glycaemic index, such as porridge, bran or muesli, may be less vulnerable to obesity. This type of breakfast, where sugars are released slowly into the bloodstream, also means children need to eat less for lunch and tend not to snack between meals.

Carrots: These nutritious vegetables are perfect for children, who often like their sweet taste. Carrot juice can also help to bind and discharge heavy metals – toxins that adults and children are exposed to in everyday living and are stored in fatty tissue.

Carrots also contain an excellent source of vitamin A, calcium, phosphorus, iron, sodium, potassium and vitamin B complex.

Calcium-rich foods: Most people automatically think of milk for calcium but there are many other foods that you can give your children. Tinned sardines, broccoli, kidney beans and cheese are sources.

Between the ages of two and seven, children need about 600mg of calcium daily to help with the strong formation of teeth and bones.

Eggs: These contain many nutrients that are crucial to the healthy growth and development of children. Not only are they rich in protein and zinc but they also contain vitamin A (helps with vision), vitamin D (aids healthy bone growth), vitamin E (prevents disease) and B12 (forms red blood cells).

They also provide iron, which is important for brain function, and lecithin, which contributes to both memory and concentration.

Kiwis: Surprisingly, kiwi fruits contain nearly twice as much vitamin C as oranges. Just one a day will provide your child with all the vitamin C they need for that day. This important vitamin cannot be stored in our bodies, so children should be encouraged to eat vitamin-C rich foods each day.

Bananas: Children need plenty of energy. A banana is an excellent energy-boosting carbohydrate and will help to sustain energy levels and concentration throughout the day.

Bananas are also rich in potassium, which can help

to counter any excess sodium in children's diet.

Whole grains: An all-round super food for kids! They supply protein for body-building, carbs for energy and fibre to assist in providing a healthy heart and digestive system. They are also a source of essential fats and various vitamins and minerals.

Always opt for whole grains over white processed foods. Much of a foodstuff's nutritional value is lost in the processing - for example, zinc, magnesium and vitamin B6 and E content.

Did You Know... ?

A 2001 survey commissioned by Haliborange found that three times as many children from the South and Midlands ate more fruit and vegetables during exam time than Northerners

And finally

Introducing your child to a healthy diet is perhaps the most important thing that you can do to have an effect on their health and well-being for the rest of their lives. You may feel daunted by the task ahead, but use this guide to start to encourage change while they are still young.

Be persistent. The taste buds on our tongue are renewed every ten days, so don't give up trying new foods out on them. If they turn something down once try a few weeks later, or in a different style.

It is also important to educate children about healthy eating and what constitutes a balanced diet. Talk to them as you prepare meals or lunchboxes and while you are doing the supermarket shopping.

Once children begin to understand why they are expected to eat their vegetables it should be easier. I'm convinced you can do it. Make just a few changes each week and, before you know it, your child will be gobbling up aubergine and asking for tofu.

Further

Updates to this guide can be found at: www.quick123.co.uk/food

On paper

Brain Food for Kids
by Nicola Graimes (Carroll & Brown, 2004)

Coping with a Picky Eater: A guide for the perplexed parent
by William G Wilkoff (Prentice Hall, 1998)

Dump the Junk: Over 300 tips to encourage children to eat healthy food
by Mary Whiting (Moonscape, 2003)

Food and You: A guide to healthy habits for teens
by Marjolijn Bijlefeld and Sharon K Zoumbaris (Greenwood Press, 2001)

The Food our Children Eat: How to get children to like good food
by Joanna Blythman (Fourth Estate, 2000)

Jamie's Dinners
by Jamie Oliver (Michael Joseph, 2004)

reading

Planet Organic: Baby and toddler cookbook
by Lizzie Vann (Dorling Kindersley, 2000)

Not on the Label:
What really goes into the food on your plate
by Felicity Lawrence (Penguin, 2004)

What are we Feeding our Kids?
by Michael F Jacobson and Bruce Maxwell (Workman, 1994)

On the web

The Food Standards Agency: **www.food.gov.uk** and **www.eatwell.gov.uk**

Food Commission: **www.foodcomm.org.uk**

The British Dietetic Association: **www.bda.uk.com**

British Nutrition Foundation: **www.nutrition.org.uk**

Consensus Action on Salt and Health: **www.hyp.ac.uk/cash**

Feed Me Better: **www.feedmebetter.com**

Hyperactive Children's Support Group: **www.hacsg.org.uk**

Just Eat More (Fruit and Veg): **www.5aday.nhs.uk**

Organix: **www.organix.com**

Think Vegetables: **www.thinkvegetables.co.uk**